WEIGHT BEARING EXERCISE FOR SENIORS WITH OSTEOPOROSIS

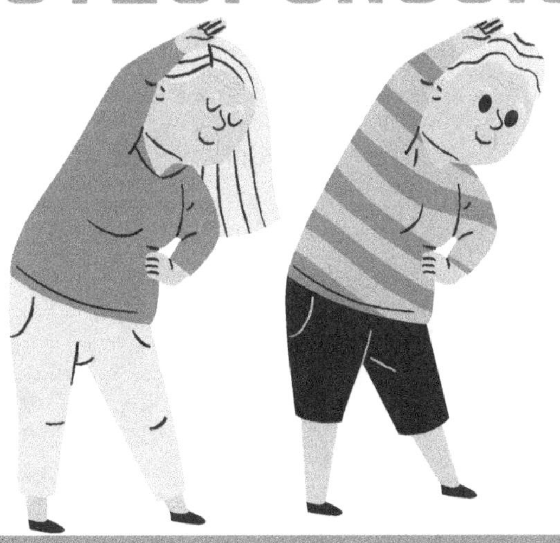

The Essential Guide to Safe and Effective Strength Training for Osteoporosis Using Low-Impact Weight Bearing Workouts to Reduce Fracture Risk

Troy Vhodes

Copyright © 2024 by Troy Vhodes

Table of Contents

Introduction

In the quiet moments of life, we often find ourselves yearning for strength, resilience, and a path to reclaim our vitality. If you're holding this book, you've already taken the first step toward a transformative journey – a journey that transcends the limitations imposed by osteoporosis, guiding you towards a life of renewed vigor and unyielding strength.

Imagine a life where every step you take is a testament to your inner power, a life where the fear of fractures fades away, replaced by the assurance of stability and mobility. This is not just a guide; it's a beacon of hope, a compass pointing towards a future where your body defies expectations and embraces the essence of vitality.

Let me share a story – a story not of the extraordinary, but of the profoundly relatable. Picture a moment in time when I, too, faced the challenges of physical limitations. The journey began with the realization that amidst the struggles of osteoporosis, there was an untapped reservoir of strength within. This guide is not just a collection of exercises; it's a narrative of triumph over adversity, a testament to the life-changing impact of safe and effective strength training.

Embark with me on a journey through the pages of "Weight Bearing Exercise for Seniors with Osteoporosis: The Essential Guide to Safe and Effective Strength Training." This isn't just about lifting weights or following a routine; it's about rewriting the story your body tells.

It's about Low-Impact Weight Bearing Workouts that not only reduce the risk of fractures but elevate your mobility to new heights.

As you dive into these pages, envision a future where every movement is a celebration of your newfound strength. Discover the joy of exercising safely, the thrill of progressing week by week, and the fulfillment of reclaiming your life from the clutches of osteoporosis.

In the following chapters, we'll explore the science behind building bone density, the art of safe and effective strength training, and the beauty of low-impact weight bearing exercises. We'll unravel the mysteries of nutrition, delve into lifestyle factors affecting bone health, and explore holistic approaches to enrich your well-being.

But before we embark on this odyssey, ask yourself: What if your journey to a stronger, more resilient you could begin today? What if this guide holds the key to sculpting a future where fractures are mere memories, and every step forward is a testament to your newfound strength?

Join me as we embark on a transformative expedition, where the destination is not just a physical state but a state of unbridled confidence and well-being. The pages ahead are not just about exercises; they are the roadmap to a life where your body defies expectations, and osteoporosis becomes a chapter of the past.

Turn the page, and let the journey begin. Your story of strength awaits.

Chapter 1
The Basics of Weight Bearing Exercises
Exploring Different Exercise Modalities

In the vibrant world of weight-bearing exercises, consider this chapter your passport to a realm where every movement is a step towards unearthing the strength that resides within. So, kick back, grab a cup of coffee, and let's delve into the exhilarating universe of muscle-building wonder.

Imagine our bodies as canvases, and weight-bearing exercises as the brushstrokes that define our strength masterpiece. In this chapter, we'll waltz through different exercise modalities, each a unique dance step in the grand choreography of building bone density and resilience.

Why dance, you ask? Well, much like a dance, weight-bearing exercises are about rhythm, coordination, and the harmonious symphony of muscle engagement. Picture it: the graceful sway of a tree pose, the rhythmic pulsing of a squat, and the elegant flow of a walking lunge – all movements intricately designed to sculpt your body into a work of art.

The Importance of Weight Bearing: Your Body's Symphony

Weight-bearing exercises aren't just about lifting things; they're about orchestrating a symphony within your bones. Your body craves the beat of impact, the rhythmic percussion that stimulates bone cells to tango and tangle, making them denser, stronger, and more resilient.

Think of it as a love story between your bones and the ground, a tale where every step, jump, or lift is a declaration of commitment to your skeletal health. And just like any epic love story, the stakes are high; fractures are the villains we aim to defeat, and mobility is the happily ever after we strive to achieve.

So, as we embark on this dance of strength, envision your body as the lead dancer, gracefully navigating the steps of weight-bearing exercises. This isn't just a workout routine; it's your body's love letter to longevity and vitality.

Ready to waltz into the world of weight-bearing exercises? Turn the page, and let the dance begin. After all, your bones are waiting for their moment in the spotlight!

Types of Weight Bearing Exercises

Welcome to the gallery of movements that will sculpt your strength, foster resilience, and redefine your journey towards better bone health. In this section, we'll explore the diverse palette of weight-bearing exercises, each stroke designed to create a masterpiece of vitality. So, let's embark on this artistic journey step by step.

Step 1: The Foundation - Weighted Walks and Marches

Our journey begins with the simplest yet incredibly effective foundation: walking. Picture this as the canvas upon which we build your skeletal masterpiece. Add a twist, and you have marches – lifting those knees to the beat of your favorite tune. These exercises form the backdrop of your routine, setting the rhythm for the entire symphony.

Step 2: The Pillars - Squats and Lunges

Now, let's introduce the pillars that support the strength of your composition – squats and lunges. Squats are the building blocks, engaging a multitude of muscles in one harmonious movement. Lunges, on the other hand, add dimension, challenging your stability and enhancing the intricacy of your bone-building tableau.

Step 3: The Spirals - Jumping and Hopping

Take a leap into the next dimension with the spirals of jumping and hopping exercises. These dynamic movements infuse energy into your routine, sending vibrations through your bones, awakening them to the call of strength. Jump, hop, and feel the spirals intertwining with the previous steps, creating a dynamic rhythm.

Step 4: The Flourishes - Step-ups and Stair Climbing

Imagine adding flourishes to your composition, step-ups and stair climbing. These movements bring elegance and complexity to your routine, targeting specific muscle groups and challenging your body to adapt to varied terrains. As you ascend and descend, your bones respond to the challenge, growing denser with each graceful step.

Step 5: The Crescendo - Resistance Training

Finally, we reach the crescendo of our weight-bearing symphony, resistance training. Whether with weights, resistance bands, or your body weight, this step adds intensity and depth to your routine. Engage your muscles against resistance, and watch as your bones respond with a resounding crescendo of strength.

In this section, we've journeyed through the fundamental steps of weight-bearing exercises – from the foundation of walks and marches to the crescendo of resistance training. Each step is a stroke on your canvas, creating a composition of strength, resilience, and bone health. Now, turn the page and let's dive deeper into crafting your personalized masterpiece. Your journey to stronger bones awaits.

Assessing Personal Fitness Levels

Embarking on a journey of strength begins with a crucial step, understanding where you stand in your fitness landscape. In this section, we'll unravel the process of assessing your personal fitness levels, ensuring a safe and tailored start to your bone-building odyssey.

Step 1: Self-Reflection - Know Your Body

Begin by looking inward. Reflect on your overall health, any pre-existing conditions, and your familiarity with physical activity. Acknowledge your strengths and be mindful of any limitations. This self-awareness sets the stage for a personalized approach to weight-bearing exercises.

Step 2: Medical Consultation - Seek Professional Guidance

Before diving into any new fitness routine, consult with your healthcare provider. They can provide valuable insights into your medical history, offer personalized recommendations, and ensure that your chosen exercises align with your overall health goals. This step is fundamental to establishing a safe starting point tailored to your unique needs.

Step 3: Mobility Assessment - Understand Your Range of Motion

Conduct a gentle assessment of your mobility. Pay attention to how freely you can move your joints, noting any areas of stiffness or discomfort. This evaluation helps identify specific areas that may require targeted attention during your weight-bearing exercises.

Step 4: Strength Inventory - Gauge Your Muscle Endurance

Determine your current strength levels by performing basic exercises without external resistance. This could include bodyweight squats, lunges, or simple balance exercises. Assess how your muscles respond, focusing on endurance and stability. Understanding your baseline strength informs the progression of your routine.

Step 5: Gradual Progression - Start Conservatively

With a clear picture of your fitness baseline, initiate your weight-bearing journey conservatively. Begin with low-intensity exercises and a manageable volume. This not only minimizes the risk of injury but also allows your body to adapt gradually. A slow and steady start sets the foundation for sustainable progress.

Step 6: Listen to Your Body - Adjust as Needed

Throughout your fitness journey, maintain an open line of communication with your body. Pay attention to how it responds to each exercise. If you experience pain, discomfort, or excessive fatigue, consider it a signal to reassess and modify your routine. Listening to your body is a key element in ensuring a safe and enjoyable exercise experience.

Step 7: Regular Reassessments - Measure Your Progress

As you progress, regularly reassess your fitness levels. This ongoing evaluation allows you to adapt your routine based on improvements, ensuring that your weight-bearing exercises continue to align with your evolving capabilities.

In this section, we've laid out a systematic approach to assessing your personal fitness levels. Each step is a crucial element in establishing a safe starting point for your weight-bearing exercise journey. Now, armed with self-awareness and professional guidance, you're ready to take the next step towards building bone density and resilience. Turn the page, and let the transformative process unfold.

Customizing Workouts for Individual Needs

One size does not fit all, especially when it comes to building strength and resilience. In this section, we'll guide you through the process of customizing your weight-bearing workouts to meet your unique needs and goals. Let's dive into the step-by-step process of tailoring your exercises for a truly personalized fitness journey.

Step 1: Define Your Objectives - Set Clear Goals

Begin by clearly defining your fitness objectives. Whether your goal is to improve bone density, enhance stability, or boost overall well-being, having a specific aim will guide the customization process. This step lays the foundation for designing a workout routine that aligns with your individual aspirations.

Step 2: Consider Your Health Status - Account for Limitations

Take into account any health considerations or limitations you may have. If you're managing specific conditions or injuries, tailor your workouts to accommodate these factors. This proactive approach ensures that your exercise routine not only enhances your fitness but also supports your overall health and well-being.

Step 3: Embrace Variety - Mix Up Your Exercises

Diversify your workout routine by incorporating a variety of weight-bearing exercises. Engaging different muscle groups and movement patterns not only prevents monotony but also ensures a well-rounded approach to strength training. This step fosters adaptability and challenges your body in various ways, contributing to a comprehensive fitness experience.

Step 4: Adapt Intensity and Volume - Listen to Your Body

Customization involves adapting the intensity and volume of your workouts based on your fitness level and progress. Gradually increase the difficulty as your strength improves, but always listen to your body. Avoid pushing too hard, too fast, and allow your routine to evolve organically, aligning with your body's capabilities.

Step 5: Incorporate Modifications - Tailor to Your Abilities

Not every exercise has to look the same for everyone. Embrace modifications that suit your abilities. Whether it's adjusting the range of motion, using support, or modifying the resistance, tailor each exercise to ensure it's challenging yet achievable for you. This adaptive approach fosters inclusivity and sustainability in your fitness journey.

Step 6: Prioritize Balance - Address Strength Disparities

Assess and address any disparities in muscle strength or flexibility. Customizing your workouts involves giving attention to areas that may be lagging behind. Incorporate exercises that target specific muscle groups or imbalances, fostering equilibrium and reducing the risk of injuries.

Step 7: Listen to Feedback - Adjust Accordingly

Pay attention to how your body responds to different exercises. If you experience discomfort, fatigue, or notice specific areas of improvement, use this feedback to fine-tune your routine. The ability to adjust and refine your workouts based on your body's signals is a key element in achieving long-term success.

Periodically review and update your workout routine. As your fitness levels evolve, so should your exercises. This ongoing customization ensures that your weight-bearing workouts remain aligned with your goals, providing a dynamic and effective fitness experience.

In this section, we've outlined a comprehensive guide to customizing your weight-bearing workouts. Each step is a crucial component in creating a tailored fitness routine that not only meets your individual needs but also evolves with your progress. Now, armed with the knowledge of customization, you're ready to sculpt a workout routine that reflects your unique strengths and aspirations. Turn the page, and let the personalized fitness journey unfold.

Chapter 2
Building Bone Density and Stability
The Science Behind Bone Health

Understanding the intricate dance between exercise, bone density, and stability is fundamental to crafting a fitness routine that truly nurtures your skeletal well-being. In this section, we'll unravel the science behind bone health, exploring how exercise influences bone density and emphasizing the crucial role of stability in managing osteoporosis.

How Exercise Impacts Bone Density

Bones, though sturdy, are remarkably responsive to the demands we place on them through physical activity. The process of bone remodeling, akin to a continuous construction and demolition project within your skeleton, is orchestrated by exercise.

When you engage in weight-bearing exercises, especially those that involve impact or resistance, you send a powerful signal to your bones. This signal stimulates the bone-forming cells, known as osteoblasts, encouraging them to produce new bone tissue. The mechanical stress applied during exercises like walking, jogging, or strength training triggers a dynamic response, leading to increased bone density over time.

The impact is most pronounced in weight-bearing exercises, where the gravitational forces transmitted through your bones during activities like walking or dancing stimulate bone-building processes. As a result, bones become denser, stronger, and better equipped to resist fractures.

This isn't just about lifting weights; it's about cultivating a relationship with your skeletal structure. By consistently engaging in activities that challenge and support bone health, you embark on a journey of fortifying the very foundation of your physical resilience.

Importance of Stability in Osteoporosis Management

Stability is the unsung hero in the realm of osteoporosis management. In the delicate dance of bone health, stability plays a central role in preventing falls and fractures, especially for those grappling with osteoporosis.

When we talk about stability, we're referring to the ability of your body to maintain balance and control during various movements. As bones become denser through exercise, stability becomes a natural byproduct. The muscles surrounding your bones, strengthened by weight-bearing exercises, act as guardians, providing essential support to prevent accidental slips and falls.

For individuals with osteoporosis, the risk of fractures is heightened, making stability a critical component of their fitness journey. Exercises that enhance balance, coordination, and core strength are pivotal. These could include activities like yoga, tai chi, or specific balance drills.

Furthermore, stability training isn't just about preventing falls; it's about fostering confidence in movement. By developing stability, you empower yourself to navigate daily activities with assurance, reducing the fear of fractures and enhancing your overall quality of life.

In summary, the science behind bone health intertwines with the art of exercise. Weight-bearing activities stimulate bone density, fortifying your skeletal framework. Concurrently, prioritizing stability becomes a cornerstone in osteoporosis management, creating a protective shield against potential fractures. Together, these elements form a powerful synergy, setting the stage for a journey towards stronger, more resilient bones. Turn the page, and let's delve deeper into the intricate tapestry of building bone density and stability.

Tailoring Exercises for Bone Building

Now that we've explored the science behind bone health, let's delve into the practical aspect of tailoring exercises specifically designed for building bone density. In this section, we'll focus on progressive training techniques tailored for seniors, ensuring a safe and effective approach to fortifying skeletal strength.

Step 1: Warm-Up

Before diving into bone-building exercises, initiate with a thorough warm-up. This could include five to ten minutes of light cardio, such as brisk walking or marching in place. Warming up increases blood flow to the muscles and prepares your body for the upcoming workout.

Step 2: Weight-Bearing Exercises

1. Bodyweight Squats:
   * Stand with feet shoulder-width apart.
   * Slowly lower your body, as if sitting back into an imaginary chair.
   * Keep your back straight, and knees aligned with your toes.
   * Rise back up to the starting position.
   * Aim for 2 sets of 10-15 repetitions.

2. Walking Lunges:
   * Take a step forward with one foot, lowering your hips until both knees are bent at a 90-degree angle.
   * Push off the front foot and bring the back foot forward.
   * Repeat on the other leg.

- Perform 2 sets of 10-12 lunges per leg.

3. Step-Ups:
  - Find a sturdy bench or step.
  - Step up onto the bench with one foot, then bring the other foot up.
  - Step back down.
  - Perform 2 sets of 10-12 step-ups on each leg.

4. Heel Raises:
  - Stand with feet hip-width apart.
  - Lift your heels off the ground, rising onto your toes.
  - Lower back down.
  - Aim for 2 sets of 15-20 heel raises.

Step 3: Resistance Training

1. Banded Leg Press:
  - Sit on a sturdy chair with a resistance band looped around your thighs.
  - Press your legs outward against the resistance.
  - Release and repeat.
  - Perform 2 sets of 12-15 repetitions.

2. Bicep Curls with Light Weights:
  - Hold a light weight in each hand, arms by your sides.
  - Curl the weights toward your shoulders.
  - Lower back down.
  - Aim for 2 sets of 12-15 repetitions.

Step 4: Cool Down

Conclude your session with a cool-down period. This could involve gentle stretching, focusing on the major muscle groups you engaged during your workout. Stretching promotes flexibility and helps prevent muscle stiffness.

Step 5: Progressive Approach

Gradually increase the intensity of your exercises as your strength improves. This could involve adding more resistance, increasing repetitions, or incorporating more challenging variations of the exercises. Consistency is key – aim for at least two to three sessions per week to experience optimal bone-building benefits.

By tailoring your exercises to include a mix of weight-bearing and resistance training, you create a comprehensive routine that supports bone health. The progressive approach ensures that you continually challenge your bones, fostering growth and resilience over time. Now, equipped with this step-by-step guide, you're ready to embark on a journey towards building stronger, denser bones. Turn the page, and let the transformative process unfold.

engaged during your workout. Stretching promotes flexibility and helps prevent muscle stiffness.

Gradually increase the intensity of your exercises as your strength improves. This could involve adding more resistance, increasing repetitions, or incorporating more challenging variations of the exercises. Consistency is key – aim for at least two to three sessions per week to experience optimal bone-building benefits.

By tailoring your exercises to include a mix of weight-bearing and resistance training, you create a comprehensive routine that supports bone health. The progressive approach ensures that you continually challenge your bones, fostering growth and resilience over time. Now, equipped with this step-by-step guide, you're ready to embark on a journey towards building stronger, denser bones. Turn the page, and let the transformative process unfold.

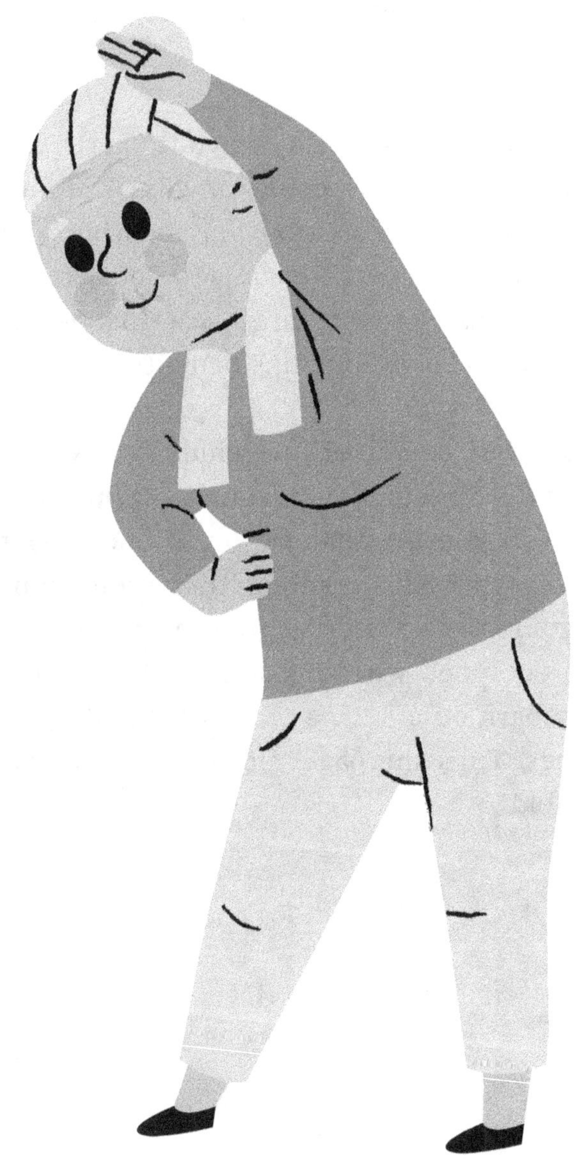

Chapter 3
Safe and Effective Strength Training Techniques
Guidelines for Safe Strength Training

Strength training is a powerful tool for building bone density and overall resilience, but safety should always be the top priority. In this section, we'll delve into essential guidelines to ensure your strength training endeavors are not only effective but, most importantly, safe. Let's explore the importance of proper form and technique while highlighting common mistakes to steer clear of.

Proper Form and Technique: The Cornerstones of Safety

1. Warm-Up Before Lifting:

Always begin with a thorough warm-up. This increases blood flow to the muscles, preparing them for the upcoming resistance.

2. Start with a Comfortable Weight:

Choose a weight that challenges you without compromising your form. If you're new to strength training, start with lighter weights and progressively increase as your strength improves.

3. Maintain Neutral Spine:

Whether you're lifting weights or performing bodyweight exercises, keep your spine in a neutral position. This minimizes stress on your back and reduces the risk of injuries.

4. Control the Movement:

Focus on controlled movements throughout the entire range of motion. Avoid relying on momentum to lift weights, as this places unnecessary strain on your joints.

5. Breathe Properly:

Don't hold your breath. Inhale during the easier part of the movement and exhale during the more challenging phase. Proper breathing ensures sufficient oxygen supply to your muscles.

6. Adapt Exercises to Your Abilities:

Modify exercises based on your individual abilities and any pre-existing conditions. If a specific movement causes discomfort, find an alternative or adjust the range of motion.

7. Proper Grip:

Maintain a secure and comfortable grip on weights or resistance bands. This enhances your control over the equipment and reduces the risk of accidents.

8. Rest Between Sets:

Allow adequate rest between sets to prevent fatigue-induced mistakes. The goal is to challenge your muscles safely, not compromise your form due to exhaustion.

Common Mistakes to Avoid: Protecting Yourself From Pitfalls

1. Ignoring Warm-Up:

Skipping the warm-up increases the risk of injuries. Always dedicate time to preparing your muscles and joints for the upcoming strength training session.

2. Lifting Too Heavy Too Soon:

Progress gradually. Lifting weights that are too heavy increases the likelihood of poor form and potential injuries. Start with manageable resistance and build from there.

3. Overlooking Posture:

Poor posture places strain on your spine and joints. Focus on maintaining proper posture throughout each exercise to optimize safety and effectiveness.

4. Neglecting Breathing Technique:

Improper breathing can lead to dizziness and compromise your form. Be mindful of your breath, and sync it with your movements.

5. Rushing Through Exercises:

Performing exercises too quickly sacrifices proper form. Take your time, ensuring each repetition is controlled and intentional.

6. Ignoring Pain:

Never ignore pain during strength training. Pain is a signal that something isn't right. If you experience persistent discomfort, consult with a healthcare professional.

7. Favoring Quantity Over Quality:

It's not about how many repetitions you can do but how well you do each one. Prioritize quality over quantity to maximize benefits and minimize risks.

8. Forgetting Cool Down:

Just as warming up is crucial, so is cooling down. Stretching post-exercise enhances flexibility and helps prevent muscle stiffness.

By adhering to these guidelines and avoiding common mistakes, you create a foundation for safe and effective strength training. Remember, your journey to stronger bones should be empowering, not compromising. Now, equipped with this knowledge, let's proceed to sculpting your strength with confidence and safety. Turn the page, and let the transformative process continue.

Incorporating Resistance: Weights, Bands, and Bodyweight

To truly enhance your strength and build robust bone density, it's time to explore the dynamic world of resistance training. This section will guide you through the incorporation of various resistance methods – weights, bands, and your own body weight. Additionally, we'll emphasize the importance of gradual progression, ensuring a steady and sustainable climb towards increased strength.

Gradual Progression for Strength: The Building Blocks

1. Begin with Bodyweight:

Start your journey with exercises that utilize your own body weight. Squats, lunges, and push-ups are excellent choices to establish a foundation of strength. This allows your body to adapt to the demands of resistance training.

2. Introduce Resistance Bands:

Resistance bands offer a versatile and accessible form of resistance. Incorporate bands into exercises like bicep curls, leg press, or lateral raises. The beauty of bands lies in their ability to provide resistance throughout the entire range of motion, engaging muscles effectively.

3. Include Dumbbells or Kettlebells:

As your strength progresses, introduce external weights like dumbbells or kettlebells. These additions amplify the challenge, especially in exercises such as squats, deadlifts, and overhead presses. Choose weights that are challenging yet allow you to maintain proper form.

4. Explore Machine-Based Resistance:

If available, consider incorporating machines that provide guided resistance. Leg press machines, cable machines, or chest press machines offer controlled resistance, making them suitable for those new to strength training.

5. Bodyweight with Added Resistance:

Advance your bodyweight exercises by adding resistance. For example, hold a dumbbell while doing squats or wear a weighted vest during lunges. This method elevates the difficulty while maintaining the convenience of bodyweight exercises.

The Importance of Gradual Progression: Nurturing Long-Term Strength

1. Avoid Rapid Increases in Intensity:

Progress should be steady, not rushed. Avoid the temptation to dramatically increase weights or resistance. Rapid jumps in intensity can lead to poor form and increase the risk of injuries.

2. Listen to Your Body:

Pay attention to how your body responds to increased resistance. If you experience persistent discomfort, consider scaling back or adjusting your approach. Consistent, moderate progression is key.

3. Periodize Your Training:

Periodization involves organizing your training into phases, alternating between periods of higher and lower intensity. This strategic approach prevents burnout and supports continuous improvement.

4. Set Realistic Goals:

Define achievable short-term and long-term goals. Celebrate small victories along the way, recognizing that building strength is a gradual and ongoing process.

5. Include Recovery Periods:

Incorporate recovery days into your routine to allow your muscles and bones time to adapt and repair. Rest is a crucial element of the progression process.

6. Regularly Reassess and Adjust:

Periodically reassess your strength levels and adjust your resistance accordingly. This ensures that your workouts remain challenging and align with your evolving capabilities.

By incorporating resistance gradually and strategically progressing your training, you lay the groundwork for sustained strength development. Whether you choose bodyweight exercises, resistance bands, or external weights, the key is to respect your body's journey toward greater resilience. Turn the page, and let's continue sculpting strength with intention and progression.

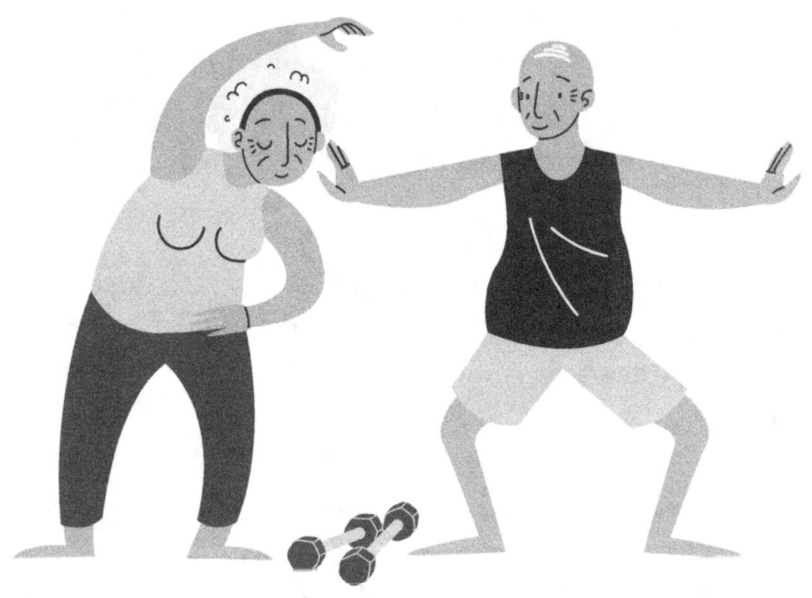

Chapter 4
Low-Impact Weight Bearing Workouts
Designing a Low-Impact Exercise Routine

When it comes to preserving joint health and minimizing stress on your body, a low-impact exercise routine is an invaluable ally. In this section, we'll explore the benefits of low-impact workouts and provide sample exercise plans to guide you towards a nurturing and sustainable fitness journey.

Benefits of Low-Impact Workouts: Embracing Gentle Strength

1. Joint-Friendly:

Low-impact exercises are gentle on your joints, making them ideal for individuals with conditions such as osteoporosis. This reduces the risk of joint strain and minimizes impact-related injuries.

2. Suitable for All Fitness Levels:

- Whether you're a beginner, returning from injury, or an active individual looking for a restorative workout, low-impact exercises are adaptable to various fitness levels. The focus is on movement and engagement rather than high-intensity impact.

3. Enhanced Stability and Balance:

Many low-impact exercises emphasize stability and balance, contributing to overall physical resilience. Improved stability is especially beneficial for seniors and those managing conditions that affect balance.

4. Reduced Muscle Soreness:

Low-impact workouts often result in less muscle soreness compared to high-impact activities. This allows for more frequent sessions and a consistent fitness routine.

5. Long-Term Sustainability:

The sustainability of a fitness routine is crucial for long-term health. Low-impact exercises are less likely to lead to burnout or overuse injuries, promoting a sustainable and enjoyable fitness journey.

Sample Exercise Plans: Building Strength with Gentleness

Plan 1: Low-Impact Cardio and Stability

1. Warm-Up:
 - Gentle marching in place - 5 minutes.

2. Cardiovascular Exercise:
 - Low-impact aerobics or brisk walking - 20 minutes.
 - Seated leg lifts or cycling - 10 minutes.

3. Stability and Balance:
 - Tai Chi or yoga for balance - 15 minutes.
 - Stability ball exercises - 10 minutes.

4. Cool Down:
 - Stretching for flexibility - 10 minutes.
 - Deep breathing or meditation - 5 minutes.

Plan 2: Low-Impact Strength Training

1. Warm-Up:
 - Arm circles and gentle jumping jacks - 5 minutes.

2. Resistance Training:
  - Bodyweight squats - 2 sets of 12-15 reps.
  - Resistance band exercises for upper body - 15 minutes.

3. Core Strengthening:
  - Seated leg lifts - 2 sets of 12-15 reps.
  - Planks or modified plank variations - 10 minutes.

4. Cool Down:
  - Gentle stretches for major muscle groups - 10 minutes.
  - Mindful relaxation - 5 minutes.

Plan 3: Low-Impact Total Body Workout

1. Warm-Up:
 - Arm swings and ankle circles - 5 minutes.

2. Total Body Exercises:
  - Swimming or water aerobics - 20 minutes.
  - Pilates or low-impact dance - 15 minutes.

3. Flexibility and Relaxation:
  - Stretching or yoga for flexibility - 15 minutes.
  - Guided relaxation or meditation - 10 minutes.

These sample exercise plans provide a variety of low-impact options to cater to your preferences and needs. Feel free to mix and match exercises based on your fitness level and enjoy the journey of gentle strength-building. Turn the page, and let the nurturing low-impact fitness routine unfold.

Adapting Workouts to Individual Mobility Levels

Every fitness journey is unique, shaped by individual mobility levels, and it's essential to design workouts that cater to a diverse range of abilities. In this section, we'll explore the art of adapting exercises to varying mobility levels, ensuring that everyone can embrace the transformative power of physical activity.

Exercises for Varied Fitness Levels: A Spectrum of Inclusivity

1. Seated Exercises:

For individuals with limited mobility or those who prefer seated workouts, exercises like seated leg lifts, seated marches, or seated arm circles provide an effective way to engage muscles and promote circulation.

2. Low-Impact Cardio Variations:

Tailor cardio workouts to accommodate different fitness levels. Brisk walking, low-impact aerobics, or water aerobics are excellent options that offer cardiovascular benefits without excessive stress on joints.

3. Chair-Assisted Workouts:

Incorporate the use of a sturdy chair for balance and support. Chair squats, chair-assisted lunges, and chair dips provide stability while targeting major muscle groups.

4. Resistance Bands for Progressive Strength:

Resistance bands are versatile tools that allow for a gradual increase in intensity.

They can be adapted for various exercises, including bicep curls, leg press, and lateral raises. Individuals can choose the level of resistance that suits their current strength.

5. Bodyweight Modifications:

Modify bodyweight exercises to accommodate different fitness levels. For example, push-ups can be done against a wall for beginners, on an incline for intermediate levels, and on the floor for those with higher strength capabilities.

6. Water-Based Exercises:

Water provides buoyancy, reducing the impact on joints. Water aerobics, swimming, or even walking in a pool are excellent options for individuals with joint concerns or limited weight-bearing capacity.

7. Adaptive Yoga and Stretching:

Yoga and stretching routines can be adapted to individual mobility levels. Seated yoga poses, gentle stretches, and the use of props like yoga blocks or straps enhance accessibility and cater to diverse abilities.

8. Customized Intervals:

Create interval workouts where participants can choose the intensity and duration of each exercise. This approach allows individuals to tailor the workout based on their fitness level, gradually progressing as they feel comfortable.

Inclusivity in Action: An Example Workout

Warm-Up:
- Gentle marching in place or seated leg swings - 5 minutes.

Cardiovascular Exercise:
- Brisk walking or low-impact aerobics - 20 minutes.
- Seated marching or low-intensity cycling for those with limited mobility - 10 minutes.

Resistance Training:
- Bodyweight squats for higher fitness levels.
- Seated leg lifts or resistance band exercises for lower fitness levels.

Balance and Stability:
- Tai Chi or standing balance exercises for those seeking challenge.
- Chair-assisted balance exercises for individuals with lower stability.

Cool Down:
- Gentle stretching for all major muscle groups - 10 minutes.
- Relaxation or meditation for mental well-being - 5 minutes.

By providing a spectrum of exercises and modifications, tailored to individual mobility levels, we create an inclusive fitness environment where everyone can participate and progress at their own pace.

This approach not only fosters a sense of empowerment but also ensures that the transformative benefits of exercise are accessible to all. Turn the page, and let the journey towards inclusive fitness continue.

Chapter 5
Personalized Exercise Plans for Seniors
Creating a Tailored Fitness Program

Embarking on a fitness journey involves more than just following a generic workout routine. It's about designing a program that is uniquely tailored to your individual needs, considering health conditions and adapting to physical limitations. In this section, we'll explore the art of crafting a fitness program that prioritizes your well-being and sets the stage for sustainable progress.

Considering Health Conditions: The Foundation of Personalized Fitness

1. Consultation with Healthcare Professionals:

Before initiating any fitness program, especially if you have pre-existing health conditions, consult with your healthcare professional. They can provide insights into specific considerations, limitations, and recommendations tailored to your health status.

2. Cardiovascular Health:

For individuals with cardiovascular conditions, low-impact aerobic exercises like walking, swimming, or cycling may be recommended. Start with shorter durations and gradually increase based on your tolerance.

3. Joint Concerns:

If joint health is a consideration, opt for low-impact exercises such as water aerobics or seated workouts. Resistance training with the guidance of a physical therapist can help strengthen supporting muscles without compromising joint health.

4. Osteoporosis or Bone Health Issues:

Focus on weight-bearing exercises to support bone health, but choose those with lower impact to reduce the risk of fractures. Activities like walking, gentle strength training, and modified yoga or Pilates can be beneficial.

5. Chronic Pain Management:

Tailor your program to manage chronic pain through exercises that emphasize flexibility, gentle stretching, and relaxation techniques. Mind-body practices like tai chi or meditation may complement your routine.

Adapting to Physical Limitations: Navigating Challenges with Creativity

1. Customized Intensity Levels:

Adjust the intensity of your workouts based on your current physical condition. Begin with lower intensities and gradually increase as your strength and endurance improve.

2. Modifications for Range of Motion:

Modify exercises to accommodate any limitations in range of motion. For example, if you have difficulty reaching overhead, perform seated arm exercises or choose alternative movements that maintain comfort.

3. Incorporating Supportive Equipment:
 Utilize supportive equipment such as resistance bands, stability balls, or chairs to enhance stability and reduce the load on certain joints. These tools can provide additional support during workouts.

4. Balancing Stability and Challenge:
 Emphasize exercises that enhance balance and stability, especially if you have concerns in these areas. Gradually introduce challenges to improve these aspects of fitness while ensuring safety.

5. Individualized Progression:
 Progress at your own pace and according to your body's response. Listen to cues such as fatigue, discomfort, or improvement, and adjust your program accordingly.

Sample Tailored Fitness Program

Warm-Up:
 Gentle joint mobility exercises - 5 minutes.

Cardiovascular Exercise:
 Low-impact walking or cycling - 20 minutes.

Resistance Training:
 Seated leg lifts with resistance bands - 2 sets of 12-15 reps.

Chair-assisted bicep curls - 2 sets of 12-15 reps.

Flexibility and Mobility:
 Modified yoga poses focusing on gentle stretches - 15 minutes.

Balance and Stability:
 Standing or seated balance exercises using a stable surface - 10 minutes.

Cool Down:
 Relaxation exercises and deep breathing - 10 minutes.

By considering health conditions and adapting to physical limitations, you create a fitness program that aligns with your unique needs. This tailored approach not only enhances your physical well-being but also fosters a positive and sustainable fitness journey. Turn the page, and let the personalized transformation unfold.

Weekly Workout Schedules

A well-rounded fitness routine involves a strategic balance of cardiovascular, strength, and flexibility exercises. In this section, we'll explore the art of crafting weekly workout schedules that optimize each component, ensuring a comprehensive and effective approach to your fitness journey.

The Importance of Balance: Cardio, Strength, Flexibility

1. Cardiovascular Exercise:

Cardio workouts elevate your heart rate, promoting cardiovascular health, endurance, and calorie burn. Engage in activities such as brisk walking, cycling, or swimming.

2. Strength Training:

Strength training builds muscle mass, enhances bone density, and contributes to overall functional fitness. Include bodyweight exercises, resistance training, or weightlifting in your routine.

3. Flexibility and Mobility:

Flexibility exercises improve joint range of motion, prevent injuries, and promote relaxation. Incorporate stretches, yoga, or Pilates to enhance flexibility and maintain joint health.

Crafting a Balanced Weekly Workout Schedule

Day 1: Cardiovascular Focus
- Brisk walking or low-impact aerobics - 30 minutes.
- Dynamic stretches to prepare for movement - 10 minutes.

Day 2: Strength Training
- Full-body strength workout incorporating bodyweight exercises or resistance bands - 30 minutes.
- Cool down with static stretches for major muscle groups - 10 minutes.

Day 3: Active Recovery or Flexibility
- Light activities such as walking, swimming, or cycling - 20 minutes.
- Emphasize flexibility with yoga or dynamic stretching - 20 minutes.

Day 4: Cardio and Strength Combination
- Interval training combining cardio bursts with strength exercises - 40 minutes.
- Incorporate resistance training for muscle engagement - 10 minutes.

Day 5: Flexibility and Mobility
- Dedicated flexibility session with static and dynamic stretches - 30 minutes.
- Gentle yoga or Pilates to enhance mobility - 20 minutes.

Day 6: Cardiovascular Endurance

- Long-duration cardio session such as hiking, cycling, or swimming - 45 minutes.
- Include intervals to vary intensity and challenge endurance - 15 minutes.

Day 7: Rest or Active Recovery

- Rest day or engage in light, enjoyable activities such as walking or gentle stretching.

Weekly Workout Schedule Tips:

1. Progressive Intensity:

Gradually increase the intensity of your workouts over the weeks. This could involve adding resistance, increasing duration, or incorporating more challenging variations.

2. Listen to Your Body:

Pay attention to how your body responds to each type of exercise. Adjust the intensity or duration based on your energy levels, soreness, and overall well-being.

3. Include Variety:

Keep your workouts interesting by incorporating a variety of exercises. This not only prevents boredom but also targets different muscle groups and movement patterns.

4. Prioritize Recovery:

Include active recovery days and ensure sufficient rest between strength training sessions. Adequate recovery is crucial for muscle repair and overall recovery.

5. Consistency is Key:

Stick to your schedule consistently. Consistency is the foundation of progress, and establishing a routine makes it easier to maintain healthy habits.

By balancing cardiovascular, strength, and flexibility exercises throughout the week, you create a holistic approach to fitness. This not only maximizes the benefits for your body but also adds variety to keep your workouts engaging and sustainable. Turn the page, and let your balanced weekly workout schedule guide you toward a fitter, healthier you.

Chapter 6
Monitoring and Adjusting Your Exercise Routine
Importance of Regular Assessments

Embarking on a fitness journey is not just about the destination; it's about the transformative process along the way. Regular assessments play a crucial role in this journey, helping you track progress and recognize warning signs. In this section, we'll delve into the significance of incorporating assessments into your fitness routine.

Tracking Progress: The Power of Measurement

1. Quantifying Achievements:
 Regular assessments provide tangible data to quantify your achievements. Whether it's an increase in strength, improved endurance, or enhanced flexibility, measurable progress boosts motivation and reinforces the value of your efforts.

2. Setting Realistic Goals:
 Assessments help you set realistic and achievable goals. By understanding your current capabilities, you can establish targets that push you slightly beyond your comfort zone, fostering continuous improvement.

3. Adapting Your Program:

As your fitness level evolves, so should your workout program. Assessments reveal areas of strength and areas that may need attention. This information allows you to adapt your routine, ensuring it remains challenging and aligned with your evolving capabilities.

4. Boosting Motivation:

Tangible evidence of progress serves as a powerful motivator. Seeing improvements, whether in increased repetitions, enhanced endurance, or greater flexibility, reinforces your commitment to the fitness journey and encourages sustained effort.

Recognizing Warning Signs: The Role of Early Detection

1. Monitoring Physical Changes:

Regular assessments help you monitor physical changes that may be indicative of underlying issues. This includes unexpected weight loss, changes in joint mobility, or alterations in muscle strength. Early detection allows for timely intervention.

2. Assessing Recovery and Fatigue:

Monitoring your body's response to workouts is essential. Assessments can reveal signs of overtraining, fatigue, or insufficient recovery. Recognizing these warning signs allows for adjustments in intensity, duration, or rest periods to prevent burnout or injuries.

3. Identifying Imbalances:

Assessments highlight muscle imbalances or weaknesses that may lead to compensatory movements. Addressing these imbalances early on can prevent the development of poor movement patterns and reduce the risk of injuries.

4. Emotional Well-Being Check:

Fitness assessments extend beyond the physical. They can serve as a checkpoint for emotional well-being. Changes in mood, energy levels, or motivation may be reflected in your performance. Recognizing these changes prompts a holistic approach to health.

Sample Assessment Components:

1. Strength Assessment:

Evaluate the maximum weight you can lift for specific exercises, such as squats, deadlifts, or bicep curls. Track changes in strength over time.

2. Endurance Assessment:

Assess your cardiovascular endurance through activities like timed walks, runs, or cycling. Note improvements in time, distance, or intensity.

3. Flexibility Assessment:

Measure joint range of motion through flexibility exercises. Track improvements in flexibility, identifying areas that may require targeted stretches.

4. Balance and Stability Assessment:
Perform balance exercises and evaluate stability. Note any improvements or areas that may need additional attention.

5. Body Composition Assessment:
Regularly measure body weight, body fat percentage, or circumferences. Recognize changes in composition and adjust nutrition or exercise accordingly.

Assessment Frequency:

1. Short-Term Assessments:
Every 4-6 weeks to capture immediate progress and adjust your program accordingly.

2. Long-Term Assessments:
Every 3-6 months to track overall fitness improvements and make more comprehensive adjustments to your fitness routine.

Conclusion:
Regular assessments form the backbone of a dynamic and effective fitness journey. By tracking progress and recognizing warning signs, you empower yourself to navigate your fitness path with informed decisions, ensuring sustainable and fulfilling results. Turn the page, and let the journey of self-discovery and improvement continue.

Making Adjustments for Continuous Improvement

Embarking on a fitness journey is a dynamic process that requires adaptability and a willingness to evolve. In this final chapter, we'll explore the art of making adjustments for continuous improvement, ensuring that your fitness routine remains aligned with your goals and evolving capabilities.

The Art of Adaptation: Why Adjustments Matter

1. Responding to Progress:

 Regular assessments provide insights into your progress. As you witness improvements in strength, endurance, or flexibility, it's essential to respond proactively. Adjustments to intensity, duration, or exercise selection can ensure that your workouts continue to challenge and stimulate growth.

2. Avoiding Plateaus:

 Plateaus are a natural part of any fitness journey. Making adjustments helps break through these plateaus by introducing variety and novelty. Whether it's changing exercises, increasing resistance, or altering workout structures, adjustments keep your body responsive to stimuli.

3. Listening to Your Body:

 Your body provides constant feedback during workouts. Pay attention to signals of fatigue, discomfort, or altered performance. Making adjustments based on these cues prevents overtraining, reduces the risk of injuries, and fosters a healthier relationship with exercise.

4. Accommodating Life Changes:

Life is dynamic, and circumstances may change. Whether it's a busy period at work, a change in schedule, or a shift in priorities, adjustments to your fitness routine ensure that it remains feasible and sustainable within the context of your life.

Key Areas for Adjustments:

1. Intensity and Volume:

Gradually increase or decrease the intensity and volume of your workouts based on your fitness goals and energy levels. This can involve adjusting the number of sets, repetitions, or resistance used in strength training, or altering the pace and duration of cardiovascular exercises.

2. Exercise Selection:

Periodically change the exercises in your routine to target different muscle groups and movement patterns. This not only prevents monotony but also ensures a more balanced and comprehensive approach to fitness.

3. Rest and Recovery:

Adapt your rest and recovery strategies based on your body's response. If you're feeling fatigued or experiencing persistent soreness, consider incorporating more rest days or adjusting the intensity of your workouts.

4. Nutritional Adjustments:

Your nutritional needs may evolve with changes in activity levels, goals, or overall health. Consider adjustments to your diet, ensuring it aligns with your fitness objectives and supports your well-being.

Sample Adjustment Scenarios:

1. Scenario 1: Increased Endurance Goals:
   If your goal shifts towards improving cardiovascular endurance, consider gradually increasing the duration and intensity of your cardio workouts. Include interval training to challenge your cardiovascular system.

2. Scenario 2: Plateau in Strength Gains:
   If you notice a plateau in strength gains, introduce variations in resistance, such as increasing weights, incorporating new exercises, or adjusting the number of sets and repetitions.

3. Scenario 3: Life Events and Schedule Changes:
   During busy periods, adapt your workout schedule to accommodate shorter, more intense sessions or focus on activities that can be easily integrated into your routine, such as quick bodyweight workouts or brief, brisk walks.

Adjustment Strategies:
1. Progressive Overload:
   Gradually increase the demands placed on your body to promote continuous improvement. This can involve adding resistance, increasing repetitions, or challenging your endurance progressively.

2. Periodization:
   Organize your training into cycles, alternating between periods of higher and lower intensity. Periodization prevents burnout, supports recovery, and facilitates ongoing progress.

3. Trial and Observation:

Experiment with adjustments and observe how your body responds. Assess the impact on your performance, recovery, and overall well-being before making more permanent changes.

4. Consultation with Professionals:

Seek guidance from fitness professionals, trainers, or healthcare providers when making significant adjustments. Their expertise can provide valuable insights and ensure that changes align with your goals and health considerations.

Conclusion: Embracing the Journey of Continuous Improvement

Making adjustments for continuous improvement is not just about refining your workouts; it's a testament to your commitment to lifelong health and well-being. As you navigate the dynamic terrain of fitness, remember that adaptation is a key ingredient for sustained progress. Embrace the journey, celebrate the victories, learn from challenges, and let the spirit of continuous improvement guide you towards a healthier, fitter you. Turn the page, and let the evolution of your fitness story unfold.

Chapter 7
Nutrition for Bone Health
Supporting Bone Health Through Diet

Bones are the foundation of our physical strength and mobility, and their health is closely tied to the nutrients we provide through our diet. In this chapter, we'll explore the crucial role of nutrition in supporting bone health, focusing on essential nutrients for osteoporosis prevention and establishing healthy eating habits for seniors.

Essential Nutrients for Osteoporosis Prevention

1. Calcium:

Calcium is a cornerstone for bone health. It contributes to bone density and strength. Include dairy products, leafy greens, fortified plant-based milk, and nuts in your diet for a calcium-rich intake.

2. Vitamin D:

Vitamin D is vital for calcium absorption. Sun exposure, fatty fish, egg yolks, and fortified foods like cereals provide this essential vitamin. Consider supplements if sun exposure is limited.

3. Magnesium:

Magnesium supports bone formation and influences the body's use of calcium. Incorporate magnesium-rich foods such as whole grains, nuts, seeds, and leafy greens into your meals.

4. Vitamin K:

Vitamin K plays a role in bone mineralization. Find it in leafy greens, broccoli, Brussels sprouts, and other cruciferous vegetables.

5. Phosphorus:

Phosphorus works alongside calcium in bone structure. Sources include dairy, lean meats, nuts, and whole grains.

6. Protein:

Protein is essential for bone and muscle health. Include lean meats, poultry, fish, beans, and dairy products to meet your protein needs.

Healthy Eating Habits for Seniors

1. Balanced Diet:
Aim for a balanced diet that includes a variety of fruits, vegetables, whole grains, lean proteins, and dairy or dairy alternatives. This ensures a diverse nutrient intake.

2. Portion Control:
As metabolism tends to slow with age, be mindful of portion sizes. Focus on nutrient-dense foods to meet your nutritional needs without excessive calories.

3. Hydration:
Stay hydrated for overall health. Water is vital for digestion, nutrient absorption, and joint health.

4. Limit Sodium and Processed Foods:

Excessive sodium can contribute to bone loss. Limit processed foods and opt for fresh, whole foods seasoned with herbs and spices.

5. Calcium-Rich Snacks:

Incorporate calcium-rich snacks like yogurt, cheese, or fortified plant-based alternatives into your daily routine to support bone health.

6. Include Omega-3 Fatty Acids:

Omega-3 fatty acids found in fatty fish, flaxseeds, chia seeds, and walnuts contribute to overall health, including bone health.

7. Moderate Caffeine and Alcohol:

Excessive caffeine and alcohol intake may interfere with calcium absorption. Enjoy these in moderation and balance them with adequate calcium-rich foods.

Sample Day of Balanced Nutrition for Bone Health:

Breakfast
- Greek yogurt with berries and a sprinkle of almonds.
- Whole grain toast with avocado.

Lunch:
- Grilled salmon or tofu with quinoa and steamed broccoli.
- Side salad with dark leafy greens.

- A handful of mixed nuts.
- Fresh fruit, such as an apple or pear.

Dinner:

- Baked chicken or lentil stew.
- Sweet potato or brown rice as a side.
- Sauteed leafy greens like kale or spinach.

Hydration:

- Drink water throughout the day.
- Include herbal teas or infused water for variety.

Conclusion: A Foundation of Wellness

Supporting bone health through diet is not only a preventive measure against osteoporosis but a fundamental aspect of overall well-being. By embracing essential nutrients and adopting healthy eating habits, you lay a solid foundation for robust bones, enhanced vitality, and a fulfilling senior lifestyle. Turn the page, and let the journey to nourish your bones unfold.

Chapter 8
Lifestyle Factors Affecting Bone Health
Impact of Smoking and Alcohol

Beyond nutrition, various lifestyle factors significantly influence bone health. In this chapter, we'll delve into the impact of smoking and alcohol consumption, explore the importance of sleep and stress management, and understand the relationship between sunlight exposure and Vitamin D synthesis.

Impact of Smoking and Alcohol

1. Smoking:

Smoking has detrimental effects on bone health. It hinders the absorption of calcium and reduces estrogen levels, leading to decreased bone density. Quitting smoking is a crucial step towards preserving bone strength and overall health.

2. Alcohol Consumption:

Excessive alcohol intake can disrupt the balance of calcium and other minerals in the body, affecting bone health. It also impairs the body's ability to absorb calcium. Moderation is key, with recommendations generally suggesting no more than one drink per day for women and two for men.

Sleep and Stress Management

1. Sleep Quality:

Adequate and quality sleep is essential for bone health. During deep sleep, the body releases growth hormone, crucial for bone regeneration. Create a conducive sleep environment, establish a regular sleep schedule, and prioritize restful sleep for optimal bone maintenance.

2. Stress Management:

Chronic stress can impact bone density and contribute to bone loss. Stress hormones, such as cortisol, may interfere with bone-building cells. Adopt stress management techniques like meditation, deep breathing, or yoga to promote overall well-being, including bone health.

Sunlight and Vitamin D

1. Sunlight Exposure:

Sunlight is a natural source of Vitamin D, a vital nutrient for bone health. Exposure to sunlight triggers the synthesis of Vitamin D in the skin. Aim for safe sun exposure, around 10-30 minutes a few times a week, depending on factors like skin tone, time of day, and location.

2. Vitamin D Intake:

In cases where sunlight exposure is limited, Vitamin D can be obtained through diet or supplements. Fatty fish, fortified dairy products, and Vitamin D supplements are common sources. Consult healthcare professionals for personalized recommendations.

Sample Strategies for Incorporating Lifestyle Changes:

1. Smoking Cessation Plan:

- Seek support from smoking cessation programs, counseling, or healthcare professionals.
- Identify triggers and develop coping strategies.
- Gradually reduce smoking or consider nicotine replacement therapy.

2. Alcohol Moderation:

- Be mindful of alcohol intake and adhere to recommended guidelines.
- Choose lower-alcohol content beverages.
- Consider alcohol-free days to reduce overall consumption.

3. Sleep Hygiene:

- Maintain a consistent sleep schedule.
- Create a relaxing bedtime routine.
- Ensure a comfortable sleep environment, including a dark and quiet room.

4. Stress Management Techniques:

- Practice mindfulness through meditation or deep breathing exercises.
- Engage in activities that bring joy and relaxation.
- Consider professional support, such as counseling or therapy.

5. Sunlight Exposure:

- Spend time outdoors during sunlight hours.
- Practice sun safety by using sunscreen and protective clothing.
- Adjust sunlight exposure based on factors like skin type and geographical location.

6. Vitamin D Supplementation:

- Consult with healthcare professionals for personalized Vitamin D recommendations.
- Take supplements as advised, especially in situations where sunlight exposure is limited.

Conclusion: A Holistic Approach to Bone Health
Understanding the impact of lifestyle factors on bone health extends the narrative beyond nutrition. By addressing smoking and alcohol consumption, prioritizing sleep and stress management, and optimizing sunlight exposure, you cultivate a holistic approach to bone health. Embrace these lifestyle changes as integral components of your journey towards maintaining strong and resilient bones. Turn the page, and let the chapters of a holistic and vibrant life unfold.

Chapter 9
Beyond Exercise – Holistic Approaches to Osteoporosis
Integrating Complementary Therapies

In the pursuit of holistic bone health, integrating complementary therapies that focus on the mind-body connection can be a transformative addition. In this chapter, we'll explore the benefits of yoga and Tai Chi, and delve into the profound impact of the mind-body connection on overall well-being.

Yoga and Tai Chi: Ancient Wisdom for Modern Wellness

1. Yoga:

Yoga is a practice that combines physical postures, breath control, and meditation. Its low-impact nature makes it ideal for seniors, promoting flexibility, balance, and stress reduction. Certain yoga poses target bone health by placing gentle pressure on bones, supporting density.

2. Tai Chi:

Tai Chi is a Chinese martial art characterized by slow, flowing movements and deep breathing. This ancient practice enhances balance, flexibility, and strength. Studies suggest that Tai Chi can contribute to bone health by improving coordination and reducing the risk of falls.

Mind-Body Connection: The Power Within

1. Stress Reduction:
Chronic stress can negatively impact bone health. Practices that cultivate the mind-body connection, such as mindfulness meditation, help manage stress levels. Reduced stress contributes to overall well-being, indirectly benefiting bone density.

2. Enhanced Body Awareness:
Mind-body practices heighten awareness of bodily sensations, movements, and postures. This heightened awareness can lead to improved posture, balance, and body mechanics, reducing the risk of falls and fractures.

3. Neurological Impact:
Mind-body practices influence the nervous system, promoting relaxation and reducing the release of stress hormones. This shift in the nervous system's state positively impacts various physiological functions, including bone metabolism.

4. Positive Hormonal Changes:
Mind-body practices may contribute to positive hormonal changes, including the release of endorphins and a reduction in cortisol levels. Endorphins, often referred to as "feel-good" hormones, contribute to an overall sense of well-being.

Incorporating Yoga and Tai Chi Into Your Routine:

1. Start Slow:

- Begin with beginner-friendly classes or videos tailored for seniors.
- Focus on mastering fundamental postures or movements before progressing.

2. Consistency Matters:

- Regular, consistent practice is key to reaping the benefits.
- Aim for at least 2-3 sessions per week, gradually increasing as you feel more comfortable.

3. Adapt to Your Abilities:

- Modify poses or movements to accommodate your comfort and physical capabilities.
- Listen to your body and avoid pushing yourself beyond your limits.

4. Combine Practices:

- Explore a combination of yoga and Tai Chi to benefit from the unique attributes of each practice.
- Consider attending classes or following online tutorials led by experienced instructors.

Mind-Body Connection Practices:

1. Mindfulness Meditation:
   - Dedicate a few minutes each day to mindfulness meditation.
   - Focus on your breath, observe sensations in your body, and cultivate a non-judgmental awareness of the present moment.

2. Breathwork (Pranayama):
   - Explore breathwork exercises that emphasize slow, deep breathing.
   - Engage in practices like diaphragmatic breathing or alternate nostril breathing.

3. Progressive Muscle Relaxation:
   - Practice progressive muscle relaxation to release tension and promote a sense of calm.
   - Gradually tense and then relax different muscle groups, starting from your toes and moving up to your head.

4. Guided Imagery:
   - Engage in guided imagery sessions that transport your mind to peaceful, serene settings.
   - Visualize healing energy flowing through your body, nourishing your bones and promoting overall health.

The Role of Medical Professionals

In the pursuit of optimal bone health, the guidance and collaboration with healthcare professionals play a pivotal role. This chapter explores the indispensable contributions of medical professionals in supporting your journey towards strong and resilient bones.

The Multifaceted Role of Medical Professionals:

1. Diagnosis and Assessment:

Medical professionals, such as orthopedic doctors, rheumatologists, or primary care physicians, play a crucial role in diagnosing and assessing bone health. Through comprehensive evaluations and diagnostic tests, they can identify conditions like osteoporosis or other bone-related issues.

2. Individualized Treatment Plans:

Once a diagnosis is established, healthcare providers craft individualized treatment plans tailored to your specific needs. This may include medication, physical therapy, and lifestyle recommendations to enhance bone health.

3. Medication Management:

In cases where medication is prescribed, medical professionals monitor its efficacy, potential side effects, and adjust treatment plans as needed. Regular follow-ups ensure that the chosen interventions align with your overall health goals.

4. Specialized Interventions:

For individuals with specific bone-related conditions, such as fractures or joint issues, orthopedic surgeons may provide specialized interventions. This could range from surgical procedures to non-invasive treatments aimed at improving bone structure and function.

Collaborating with Healthcare Providers: A Synergistic Approach

1. Open Communication:

Establish open and transparent communication with your healthcare team. Share your concerns, goals, and any changes in your health or lifestyle that may impact your bone health.

2. Regular Check-ups:

Schedule regular check-ups with your primary care physician or specialists involved in your bone health care. These check-ups allow for ongoing assessment, adjustments to treatment plans, and the early detection of any changes in your condition.

3. Engage in Shared Decision-Making:

Actively participate in shared decision-making with your healthcare providers. Discuss treatment options, potential risks and benefits, and express your preferences. This collaborative approach ensures that your care aligns with your values and priorities.

4. Educational Resources:

Seek educational resources from your healthcare providers to enhance your understanding of bone health. Knowledge empowers you to make informed decisions about your care and lifestyle.

5. Multidisciplinary Approach:

Embrace a multidisciplinary approach to bone health. Work with a team that may include orthopedic specialists, physical therapists, nutritionists, and mental health professionals. This holistic perspective addresses the various facets of bone health.

Sample Collaborative Approach:

1. Initial Assessment:
   - Visit your primary care physician for an initial assessment of bone health.
   - Undergo diagnostic tests, such as bone density scans, to evaluate bone density and identify any existing conditions.

2. Specialist Consultations:
   - If necessary, consult with specialists such as orthopedic doctors or rheumatologists for further evaluation.
   - Discuss treatment options, potential interventions, and establish a collaborative care plan.

3. Medication Management:
  - If medication is prescribed, work closely with your healthcare provider to understand its purpose, potential side effects, and proper administration.
  - Schedule regular follow-ups to monitor the medication's impact on your bone health.

4. Physical Therapy and Rehabilitation:
  - Engage in physical therapy sessions if recommended by your healthcare team.
  - Collaborate with physical therapists to improve strength, flexibility, and overall bone health.

5. Lifestyle Modifications:
  - Implement lifestyle modifications based on recommendations from healthcare providers.
  - Regularly update your healthcare team on changes in your diet, exercise routine, or any other lifestyle factors.

6. Mental Health Support:
  - Recognize the connection between mental health and overall well-being, including bone health.
  - Seek mental health support if needed, collaborating with professionals who understand the interplay between mental and physical health.

Conclusion: A Unified Path to Bone Health
Collaborating with healthcare professionals creates a unified path towards achieving and maintaining optimal bone health.

Conclusion

As you reach the final chapter of this comprehensive guide on weight-bearing exercises for seniors with osteoporosis, I invite you to reflect on the transformative journey we've embarked upon together. Your commitment to understanding and nurturing your bone health is a testament to your resilience, dedication, and the profound importance you place on your well-being.

Throughout these pages, we've explored the intricacies of weight-bearing exercises, delving into the science behind bone health, uncovering the benefits of complementary therapies, and understanding the crucial role of healthcare professionals. You've gained insights into nutrition, lifestyle factors, and the powerful mind-body connection, all woven into a tapestry of holistic well-being.

As you stand at the intersection of knowledge and action, consider this not just a guide but a companion on your path to vibrant bone health. You've learned that building and maintaining strong bones is not a singular task but a harmonious orchestration of various elements – from physical activities to mindful practices, from nutritional choices to collaborative healthcare partnerships.

Your journey doesn't conclude with these pages; it extends into the choices you make daily, the exercises you embrace with enthusiasm, the nourishment you provide your body, and the mindful moments that contribute to your overall vitality. Seize each opportunity to implement the wisdom gained, adapt to your evolving needs, and celebrate the progress, both big and small.

Remember, the journey to vibrant bone health is not a destination but a continuous exploration. Stay curious, stay committed, and stay connected – to your body, to the guidance of healthcare professionals, and to the vibrant community of individuals on a similar quest for wellness.

As you turn the final page, carry forward the empowerment that comes from understanding your body and its magnificent capabilities. May the knowledge within these chapters be a source of inspiration, guiding you towards a life filled with strength, resilience, and the joy of moving freely.

Embrace your journey with gratitude, cultivate a spirit of curiosity, and revel in the strength you are nurturing within. Your commitment to vibrant bone health is a gift to yourself – a gift that keeps on giving as you savor the richness of a life well-lived.

Thank you for entrusting me to be a part of your journey. Here's to your vibrant bone health and the chapters of wellness that lie ahead.